Legal & Disclaimer

The information contained in this book is not designed to replace or take the place of any form of medication or professional medical advice. The information in this book has been provided for educational and entertainment purposes only.

The information contained in this book has been compiled from sources deemed reliable, and it is accurate to the best of the Author's knowledge. However, the Author cannot guarantee its accuracy and validity so cannot be held liable for any errors or omissions. Changes are periodically made to this book. You must consult your doctor or get professional medical advice before using any of the suggested remedies, techniques, or information in this book.

Upon using the information contained in this book, you agree to hold harmless the Author from and against any damages, costs and expenses, including any legal fees, potentially resulting from the application of any of the information provided by this guide. This disclaimer applies to any damages or injury caused by the use and application, whether directly or indirectly, of any advice or information presented, whether for breach of contract, tort, negligence, personal injury, criminal intent, or under any other cause of action.

You agree to accept all the risks of using the information presented inside this book. You need to consult a professional medical practitioner in order to ensure you are both able & healthy enough to participate in this program.

Contents

Introduction

Are you interested in following the bodybuilding diet? Then you are making one of the best decisions for your body and overall health. It is because this diet plan aids in reducing excess body fat and building muscles. It puts more emphasis on protein-rich foods, as well as those foods rich in complex carbs, like cereal, whole-grain bread, and pasta.

A good bodybuilding diet plan consists of its one major component - a strength building exercise you have to do regularly. It requires you to stick to a workout routine for 3 to 7 days every week that is often composed of cardio and weightlifting exercises.

Just like your workout, your daily diet also plays a vital role in ensuring that you get the results of your bodybuilding exercises; hence, the need to follow a bodybuilding diet. If you are unsure how to start, then the rule of thumb is to eat the right and healthy kinds of food and make sure to stick to the appropriate amounts.

By doing that, you can supply your muscles with all the nutrients needed for them to recover from your workouts while supporting their growth. To guide you in your journey towards sticking to a bodybuilding diet, this e-book has been created. It contains some of the things you have to know about bodybuilding diet.

It also covers some recipes that are safe to include in your bodybuilding diet plan. With all the information here, you have an assurance that you can achieve your goal in terms of fitness and health.

Chapter 1 - Benefits of Bodybuilding

Bodybuilding is a popular technique implemented by those who want to bulk up and look fit. In most cases, it focuses more on building your muscles by combining proper nutrition and weightlifting. Some consider bodybuilding as a lifestyle as it requires them to spend time in and out of the gym.

To ensure that you get the results you want from bodybuilding, it is crucial to focus on your diet aside from your regular workouts. It is because eating the wrong foods can have a negative impact on your target goals. By combining proper bodybuilding workouts with proper diet, you have a hundred percent assurance that you will enjoy the following benefits:

Improves body health

One incredible advantage of bodybuilding is that it can significantly improve the health of your body. It can lessen your risk of suffering from major ailments, like coronary heart disease. This lifestyle can have a positive impact on your joints, bones, and muscles. It can strengthen your muscles and make them more flexible.

It allows you to get engaged in physical activities, like aerobic exercises and weight training that lessen your risk of dealing with obesity, high cholesterol, and high blood pressure. Furthermore, it can prevent issues, like arthritis and osteoporosis. With the many things it can do for your body, it is safe to say that bodybuilding can work wonders on your health.

Improves mental health

Bodybuilding can also contribute to boosting your mental well-being and health. By doing aerobic exercises and weight training regularly, you can lessen your risk of suffering from stress, depression, and anxiety. You can even expect it to help in boosting your confidence and self-esteem.

It does so once you were able to build a positive image of yourself, which tends to happen once you start losing weight or notice your body becoming stronger and leaner. The regular bodybuilding routines you do also contribute to improving your mood.

You will also notice a great improvement in your ability to deal with negative emotions once you start bodybuilding. It clearly indicates that your mental health is gaining benefits from your routines.

Develops motor control

Another great advantage of bodybuilding is that it aids in developing motor control, which is necessary for allowing your central nervous system to regulate your movements. Motor control is necessary because it serves as the foundation that supports all forms of exercise. Once you develop proper motor control, it will be easier for you to advance to more complex exercises and activities.

Helps make you stronger

Bodybuilding also has the advantage of strengthening your muscles. It lets you develop muscular strength, which is essential in doing certain activities, like lifting things and transferring them from one place to another. It can also strengthen your bones and ligaments. With stronger bones, ligaments, and muscles, you will have no problems doing your regular and daily routines.

Mentioned in this chapter are just a few of the many benefits that you can obtain from bodybuilding. Considering all the benefits indicated here, it is safe to say that bodybuilding is not just designed to build and strengthen your muscles but also to improve your overall health, fitness, and wellness. Just make sure to pair your bodybuilding exercises with the appropriate diet to maximize its results.

Chapter 2 – Essential Components of the Diet Plan of Bodybuilders

A bodybuilding diet will always have one goal – to help those who stick to it build muscle while reducing their body fat. One thing you should remember about this diet plan is that it focuses more on protein-rich and complex carb-rich foods. Among these are cereal, pasta, and whole-grain bread.

Although you can find several versions of this diet plan, you have to remember that one consistent component of it is a strength-building exercise you have to do regularly. Also, remember that you can only maximize the positive effects of a bodybuilding diet if you learn more about macronutrients – the three major groups of nutrients that the foods in this diet plan can provide you. These are proteins, fats, and carbohydrates.

If you want to build a great physique through bodybuilding, then you also have to make wise food choices consistently. That way, you can stick to the correct amount and level of quality for such nutrient groups.

Protein

Protein is always considered as a key nutrient for those who are aiming to build muscles, so it is a vital component in your bodybuilding diet. If the protein you take in is not enough, then you will have a hard time building muscle even if you dedicate a lot of time and effort in training.

That said, you have to focus on including foods rich in protein in your meals. Among the best sources of protein are eggs, fish, chicken, and lean meat. You also have to know the exact amount of protein your body needs, so you will be able to supply it with the right amounts.

How Much Protein Do You Need?

Note that regardless if your goal is to become muscular or lean or gain muscle mass, you can compute your protein needs by multiplying 2.5 to 3 grams of protein for every kilogram of body weight daily. For instance, if you are into bodybuilding and your bodyweight for the day is 75 kilograms, then multiply this by 2.5 to 3. The result, which is 187.50 to 225, is the number of high-quality protein (in grams) that you need to take per day.

Carbohydrates

It is also important for your body to get a good supply of carbohydrates if you want to gain the best results from bodybuilding. One thing that you have to take note of about carbs is that they can either be complex or simple. It is crucial for your bodybuilding diet to have both the complex and simple carbs to get the best results from it.

Complex carbs are known for having a chemical structure consisting of at least three sugar. You can expect these carbs to supply you with sustainable energy. On the other hand, simple carbs have a chemical structure consisting of only one to two sugars. You can expect these carbs to supply you with energy quickly, although it will only last for a short time.

For your bodybuilding diet to work favorably, it is advisable to add more complex carbs into it. You have to eat foods rich in complex carbs throughout the day if you are into bodybuilding. The best sources of complex carbs are whole grain bread, beans, cereal, and pasta. You can also get this type of carbs from most veggies.

You also need to eat simple carbs but do it right after your workout. Doing that will support the quick repair and recovery of your muscles. You can supply your body with simple carbs by including some fruits in your diet. Make sure that you also consume some sugary foods and drinks, like sports drinks, juice, and candies every now and then.

How Many Carbs Do You Need?

The question now is, how much carbs should you consume every day? If you intend to gain muscle mass, then it is highly recommended to supply your body with around 4 to 5 grams of carbs for every kilogram of body weight daily. Say, for example, you weigh 75 kilograms. You have to multiply it by 4 to 5 grams. This means that you will need around 300 to 375 grams of high-quality carbs daily.

If your goal is to build lean muscles and remove fat, then you can multiply your body weight by 1 to 2 grams. Using the same weight in the previous example, which is 75 kg., you will need around 75 to 150 grams of carbs daily to get the lean muscle mass and fat reduction you are aiming for.

Fats

Similar to carbs and proteins, you also need fats to keep your body healthy. However, make sure that you eat the right kinds of fat and at the right amount. It is because eating the wrong kind of fat excessively can lead to several health issues that can affect you for the long term, like heart disease and obesity.

Fats are available in either solid form, like fat layers in red meat and butter, or liquid form, such as vegetable oil. Just like carbs, certain kinds of fat are essential for your body, which is why you need to include them in your diet. Among these essential fats are those present in foods, such as avocado, seeds, nuts, and a few vegetable oils, like flaxseed and olive oils.

Some types of animal fat, such as fish oil, are also rich in essential fatty acids, like Omega-3 and Omega-6. With their importance, you need to make sure that some foods in your bodybuilding diet consist of fat. It is necessary to get a moderate supply of these foods every day to keep yourself healthy.

The fact that healthy and essential fats serve as vital components in your cell wall structure also makes them necessary in constructing new muscle cells. Just make sure that you also limit and avoid unhealthy fats, like the saturated ones that are usually found in animal meats.

Calorie Requirements and Macronutrients

For those who are into bodybuilding, their primary objectives include increasing muscle mass during the bulking phase and reducing body fat during the cutting phase. This means you need to have a higher consumption of calories during the bulking phase compared to your calorie intake in the cutting phase.

To determine the specific number of calories you need, weigh yourself thrice a week at the very least. You also need to record the foods you eat. If possible, use a calorie tracking app to record them. If your weight remains the same, then the number of calories you have to take every day can be referred to as your maintenance calories. It means that you do not lose nor gain weight. You only maintain it.

If that's the case, it is highly recommended to raise your calorie consumption by 15 percent once you are in the bulking phase. Once you begin to transition from the bulking to the cutting phase, lessen your maintenance calories by 15 percent.

Adjust your calorie consumption depending on the weight you gain or lose during the bulking and cutting phases, respectively. Do the adjustments monthly to ensure that they are in accordance with your weight changes.

Upon establishing your required number of calories every day, it is easy to identify your macronutrient ratio. It refers to the ratio of your carbs, protein, and fat consumption. As a rule, it is highly recommended for your daily calorie intake to consist of 30 to 35 percent protein, 55 to 60 percent carbs, and 15 to 20 percent fat.

Now that you know the major components of a bodybuilding diet as well as how to determine your calorie and nutrition requirements, it is time to create your own meal plans. Make sure to choose those recipes that you can quickly and easily prepare. The next chapters of this book will cover some easy-to-prepare recipes that you can cook or prepare within just 30 minutes or less.

Chapter 3 – 6 Easy and Quick 30-minute Breakfast Recipes for Bodybuilding

Pumpkin Omelet

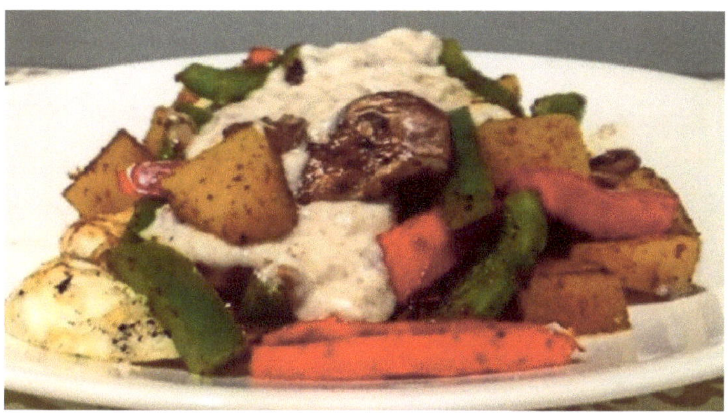

Ingredients for the Omelet:

- 5 egg whites
- ¼ cup pumpkin (cut into 1-inch cubes)
- ¼ cup each of red bell pepper, green bell pepper, and mushrooms (all sliced)
- ½ tbsp. each of paprika and chili powder

Ingredients for the Peanut Sauce:

- 2 tbsps. plain Greek yogurt (non-fat)
- 1 tbsp. peanut butter

Instructions:

1. Put the pumpkin in a medium pot then boil it until it becomes tender. This usually takes around ten minutes.
2. While waiting for the pumpkin to boil, sauté the veggies.
3. Get another pan and set it over medium heat. This is where you should cook the egg whites separately.
4. Mix pumpkin with the sautéed veggies. Add the paprika and chili powder.
5. Prepare the peanut sauce in a small bowl by mixing the two ingredients together.

6.   Get the veggie mixture then add a scoop of it on top of the egg whites. Top it further with the prepared peanut sauce.

7.   Serve.

Nutrition Facts:

Calories: 251

Protein: 27 grams

Carbs: 15 grams

Fat: 9 grams

Cauliflower Hash Browns

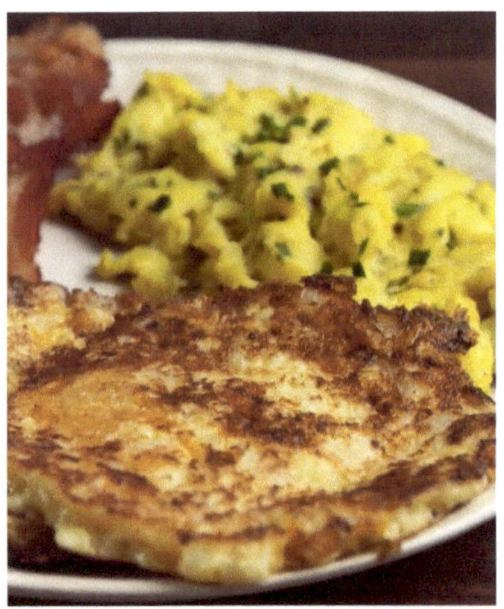

Ingredients:

- 1 whole egg
- 8 ounces cauliflower (chopped)
- 3 cups spinach
- 1 tsp. salt
- 1 finely chopped shallot
- 1 tbsp. white vinegar
- 2 eggs
- 1 tsp. lemon juice

Instructions:

1. Use your food processor or cheese grater to grate the cauliflower.
2. Mix the grated cauliflower, one egg, salt, and shallot together. Leave it for around five minutes.
3. Heat some olive oil in the already heated skillet. Spread the mixture containing the cauliflower on the skillet thinly.
4. Let the cauliflower sear using medium-high heat until it becomes brownish. This should take around 4 to 5 minutes. You should then flip it carefully, so you can sear the other side.
5. Boil one pot of water together with the white vinegar. Crack the eggs into the boiled water then cook through a gentle simmer for a couple of minutes.
6. The next step is to prepare a pan where you can wilt the spinach using one squeeze of lemon and a bit of water. Use salt to season it.
7. Once done, you can serve the hash browns plated with the poached eggs and the wilted spinach.

Nutrition Facts:

Calories: 242

Carbs: 23 grams

Protein: 19 grams

Fat: 8 grams

Spinach Omelet with Parmesan and Chives

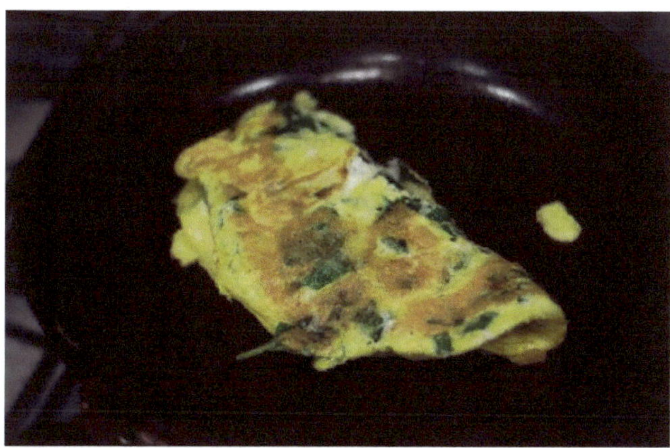

Ingredients:

- 3 eggs (beaten)
- ¼ cup cooked spinach
- 2 tbsps. each of chives (chopped), low-fat parmesan cheese, and skim milk

Instructions:

1. Get a small bowl and beat the eggs together with the egg whites and milk in there.
2. Prepare a non-stick pan and drop some olive oil into it. Set the pan over medium-high heat.
3. Add chives and the prepared egg mixture to the pan. Wait for the eggs to start solidifying then pull them at the center. Tilting the pan should be the next step, allowing any raw egg to run outside. Continue doing it until you notice that the eggs are already cooked.
4. Add the parmesan and spinach.
5. Slide the eggs slowly and gently to the pan's edge. Fold the omelet gently with the help of a spatula.
6. Cook each side briefly prior to plating and serving this dish.

Nutrition Facts:

Calories: 120

Protein: 9 grams

Fat: 7 grams

Carbs: 5 grams

Broiled Grapefruit

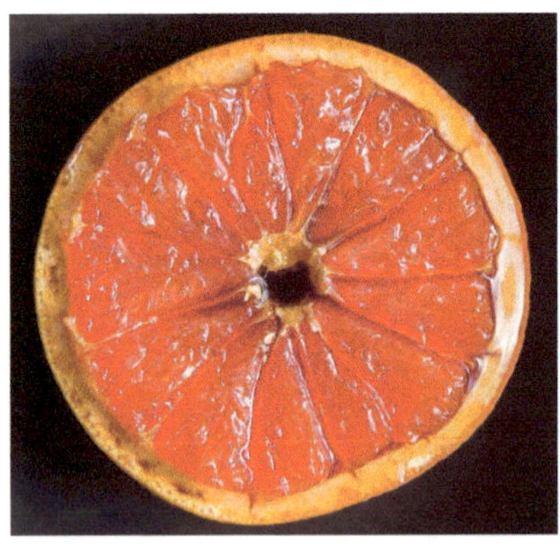

Ingredients:

- 2 grapefruits
- 1/8 tsp. each of lemon zest and vanilla extract
- 2 tbsps. honey
- 1 tsp. coconut oil
- 1 pinch sea salt

Instructions:

1. Get the grapefruits and slice them in half.
2. Separate the fruit from the rind. However, be extra careful not to remove the fruit when doing this.
3. Mix honey, vanilla, and honey in a bowl. Brush each halved grapefruit using this mixture.
4. Get a baking sheet where you can arrange the grapefruits. You should then broil the grapefruits in your oven for around 6 minutes.
5. Take the broiled grapefruits out of the oven then sprinkle it with the lemon zest and sea salt before serving.

Nutrition Facts:

Calories: 174

Carbs: 36 grams

Fat: 3 grams

Protein: 1 gram

Bacon and Egg Sandwich

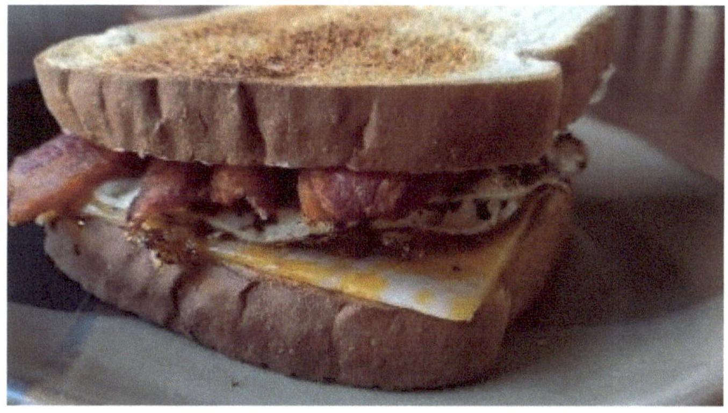

Ingredients:

- 2 slices of whole-grain bread
- 1 whole egg
- 1 slice of bacon
- 1 slice medium-sized tomato (should be around one-fourth-inch thick)
- ½ of skinless and deseeded avocado
- 1 cup spinach
- 2 slices of Colby cheese

Instructions:

1. Cook eggs depending on your preference. It could be fried, scrambled, or poached.
2. Toast the bread until it turns to golden brown. Put the eggs on one toasted bread.
3. After that, lay the two slices of cheese over the eggs. Follow the cheese with bacon and spinach. You should also add the tomato and avocado in the same order.
4. Top it with the second toasted bread. Enjoy this sandwich while it is still hot.

Nutrition Facts:

Calories: 655

Carbs: 40 grams

Fat: 39 grams

Protein: 36 grams

Cranberry and Almond Oatmeal

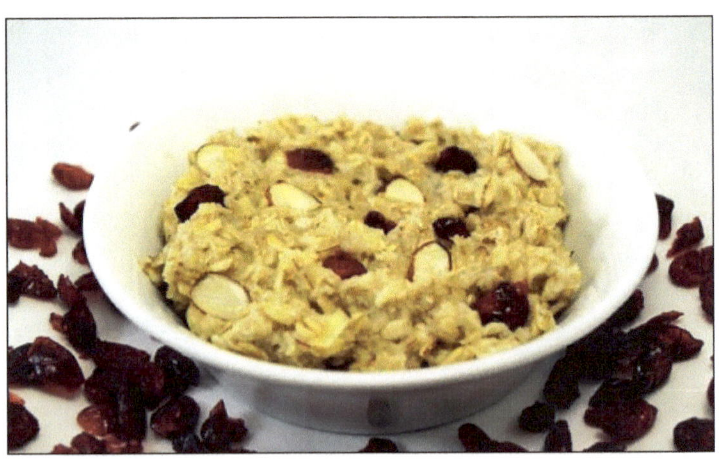

Ingredients:

- 3 tbsps. cranberries (dried)
- ¾ cup rolled oats
- 1 cup of water
- 1 and ½ scoop of vanilla whey protein powder

Instructions:

1. Mix the rolled oats, cranberries, and water in one bowl.
2. Microwave this mixture for around one to two minutes. Stir the mixture and let it rest for around a minute.
3. Add the almonds and protein powder. Serve.

Nutrition Facts:

Calories: 745

Carbs: 80 grams

Protein: 50 grams

Fat: 25 grams

Chapter 4 – 6 Easy and Quick 30-Minute Lunch Recipes for Bodybuilding

Cheesy Beef Pasta

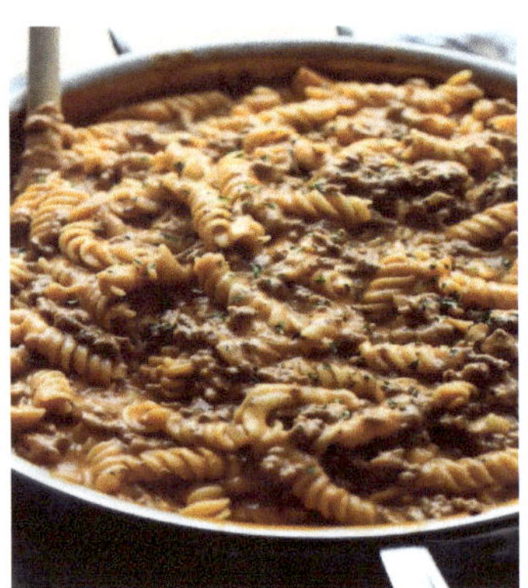

Ingredients:

- ½ lb. lean ground beef
- 2 minced garlic cloves
- 1 diced onion (or around one cup of it)
- ½ tsp. each of oregano and basil (dried)
- 1 chopped small zucchini
- ¼ tsp. hot red pepper flakes
- 1 24-oz. jar tomato-based pasta sauce
- 2-oz. or around ½ cup cheddar cheese (shredded)
- 12-oz. or around 4 cups rotini pasta
- 6-oz. or around 1 and ½ cup mozzarella cheese (shredded)

Instructions:

1. Prepare a large skillet and set it over medium-high heat. Place garlic, zucchini, onion, and beef in there and cook until you notice that the meat is already brownish in color and is broken down in pieces. After that, you should drain excess fat.
2. Mix in the basil, pasta sauce, red pepper flakes, and oregano. Simmer and cook using medium-low heat for around 15 minutes.

3.   While simmering, begin cooking the pasta based on the directions in its package.
4.   Once done, drain the pasta then pour the sauce cooked in the skillet. Add the cheese. Cover the pan until the cheese melts.
5.   Serve.

Nutrition Facts:

Calories: 507

Carbs: 81 grams

Protein: 26 grams

Fat: 9 grams

Shredded Chicken Salad

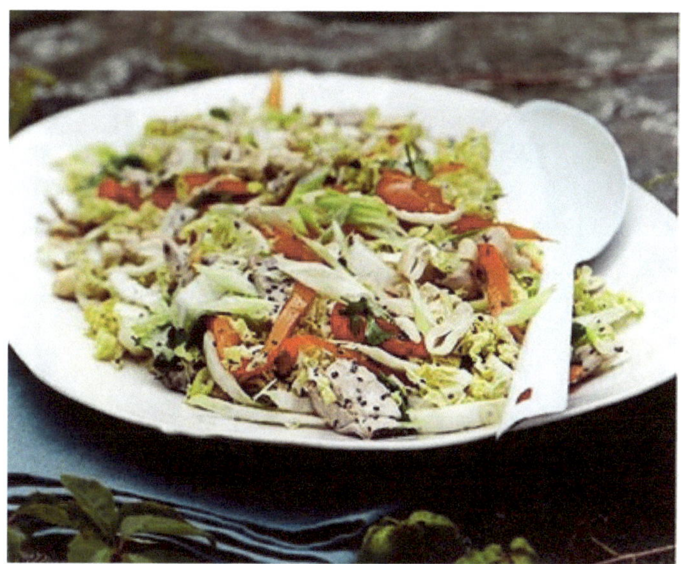

Ingredients:

- 4 tsps. ginger (freshly grated)
- 3 tbsps. chicken broth
- 2 tsps. fresh lime juice
- 1 tbsp. tamari
- 1 small seeded and diced red chili pepper
- 2 cups Napa cabbage (thinly sliced)
- 8 ounces chicken breast (cooked and shredded)

- 1 cup daikon radish (matchstick-sliced)
- 1 diagonally and thinly sliced green onion

Instructions:

1. Whisk ginger, chicken broth, fresh lime juice, tamari, and red chili pepper together in a bowl.
2. Add the radish, cabbage, and chicken. Toss the ingredients to mix well.
3. Sprinkle some green onions on top of the salad, then serve.

Nutrition Facts:

Calories: 234

Protein: 37 grams

Carbs: 9 grams

Fat: 7 grams

Avocado and Poached Egg Toast

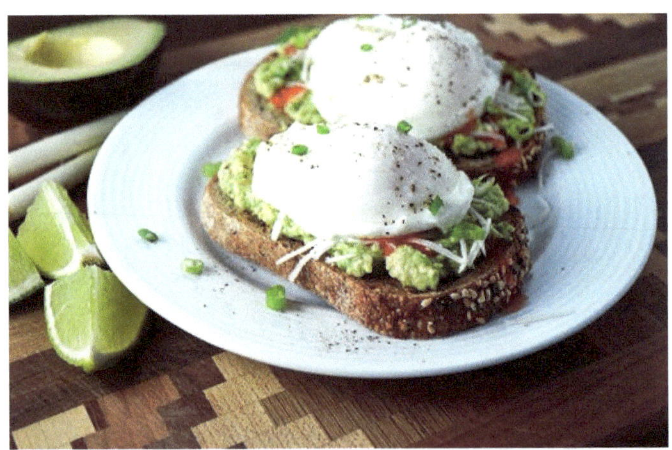

Ingredients:

- 2 whole-grain bread slices
- 2 eggs
- 2 tbsps. Parmesan cheese (shaved)
- 1/3 of an avocado
- Fresh herbs (ex. basil, thyme, or parsley)
- Some salt and pepper
- Heirloom tomatoes (quartered)

Instructions:

1. Add water to a pot. The water should be enough to cover eggs once you let them lay at the bottom of the pot. Let the water boil.
2. Get two lids of mason jars and drop their outer metal rims into the pot. They should lay flat at the bottom. Once the water boils, turn the heat off. Crack the eggs gently and carefully into the rims. Poach the eggs for around five minutes with the pot covered.
3. While you are cooking the eggs, you should start toasting the bread. Smash avocado on each toasted bread.
4. Lift the poached eggs from the water using a spatula. Pull each egg gently from the rim then put it on top of each toast.
5. Top each toast with salt, fresh herbs, pepper, and Parmesan cheese. Serve the toast together with the tomatoes.

Nutrition Facts:

Calories: 393

Carbs: 30.1 grams

Protein: 23.3 grams

Fat: 20.4 grams

Shrimp Pasta

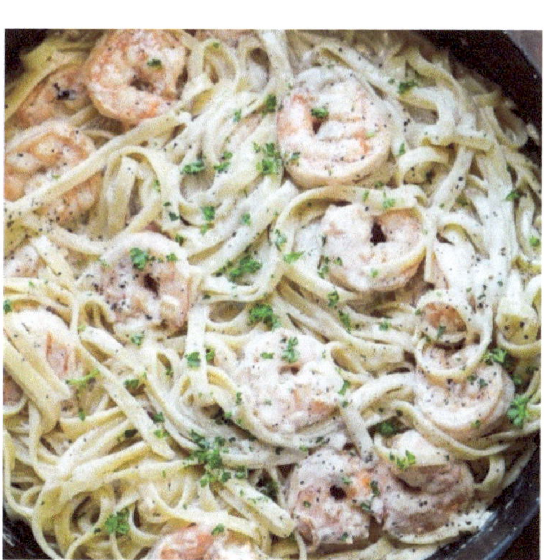

Ingredients:

- 15 small, peeled, and deveined shrimps
- ¾ cup whole-wheat pasta spaghetti

- 4 tbsps. Italian dressing
- ½ cup broccoli
- 1 cup red bell pepper (chopped and sliced)
- 1 oz. parmesan cheese (low-fat)

Instructions:

1. Boil water in a pot then cook the pasta in there based on the package instructions.
2. Heat half of the salad dressing (around 2 tbsps.) in a pan. Add the broccoli, shrimp, and peppers. Toss the ingredients then stir-fry lightly for around 2 to 3 minutes. Add the remaining salad dressing then toss again.
3. Pour this over the cooked pasta. Mix well then top with the Parmesan cheese. Serve.

Nutrition Facts:

Calories: 124

Carbs: 20 grams

Protein: 6 grams

Fat: 2 grams

Spinach, Avocado, and Bacon Salad

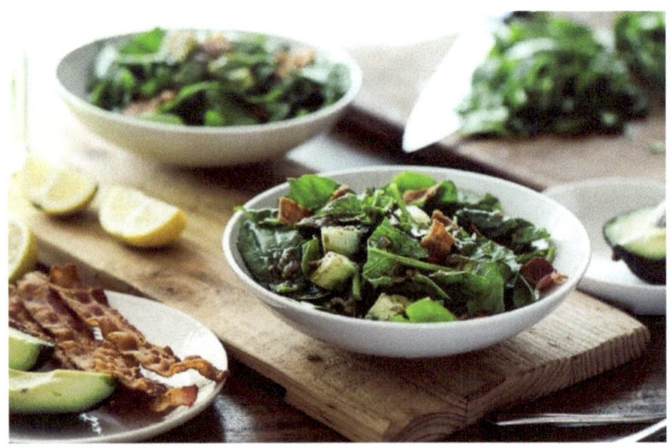

Ingredients:

- 4 cups spinach
- 3 ounces of turkey bacon
- 1 tbsp. olive oil
- 1 avocado

Instructions:

1. Heat a skillet then cook turkey bacon in there until it becomes crispy.
2. Take the skin out of the avocado. After that, you should cut it until it forms a few slices of around one-fourth-inch thick.
3. Mix spinach, avocado, and lemon juice by hand. Do the mixing until you notice that the avocado is already mashed together with the spinach.
4. Toss the cooked turkey bacon. Serve.

Nutrition Facts:

Calories: 407

Carbs: 25 grams

Protein: 24 grams

Fat: 23 grams

Tuna Burger

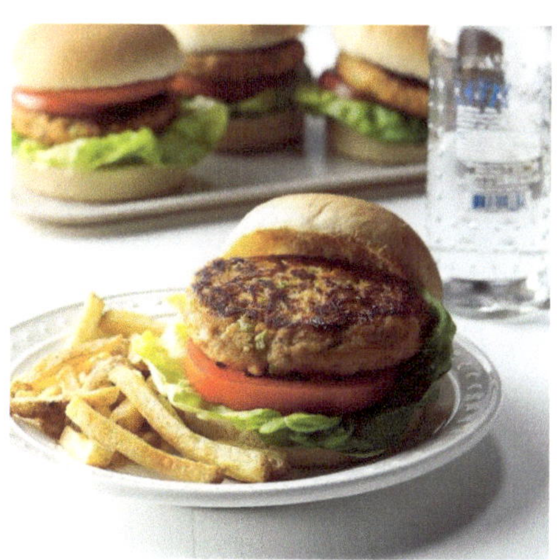

Ingredients:

- 4 cans canned tuna – Make sure to drain it before using.
- 4 tbsps. mayonnaise (fat-free)
- 1 cup panko bread crumbs (whole-wheat)
- 1 tbsp. garlic powder
- ½ cup onions (chopped)
- ¼ cup sunflower seeds

Instructions:

1. Place the drained tuna fish in a bowl. Mix it with other ingredients. Blend well.
2. Put a skillet over medium heat and let it warm a bit. While waiting for the skillet to get warm, form the mixed ingredients in the bowl into a few patties.
3. Cook the patties in the heated skillet for around five minutes per side or until they become brown and crispy.
4. Serve it as is or by garnishing it like a burger.

Nutrition Facts:

Calories: 296

Protein: 45 grams

Carbs: 22 grams

Fat: 3 grams

Chapter 5 – 6 Easy and Quick 30-Minute Dinner Recipes for Bodybuilding

Grilled Chicken Skewers

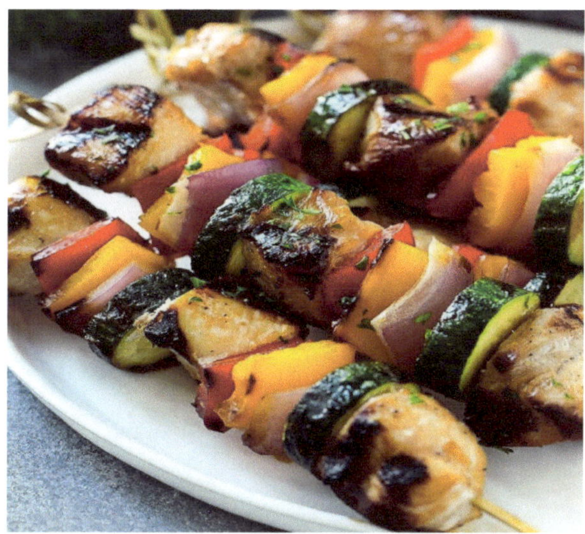

Ingredients:

- 2 pcs. chicken breast – Cut them into small pieces (about one inch each).
- 1 sliced lemon
- Juice from 1 lemon
- 2 tbsps. olive oil
- 2 minced garlic cloves
- 1 tbsp. mustard (ground)
- ¼ cup finely chopped whole basil leaves
- Some salt and pepper

Instructions:

1. Preheat your grill by setting it to medium-high heat.
2. Make the skewers by alternating one chicken cub with one slice of lemon. Fold it in half.
3. Mix garlic, basil, mustard, olive oil, salt, pepper, and lemon juice together.
4. Brush this mixture over each skewer. Make sure to cover both sides.
5. Once done, you can start grilling them using medium-high heat. The rule of thumb is to grill it for around four minutes per side. Serve.

Nutrition Facts:

Calories: 233

Protein: 31 grams

Fat: 11 grams

Carbs: 4 grams

Mustard Baked Salmon

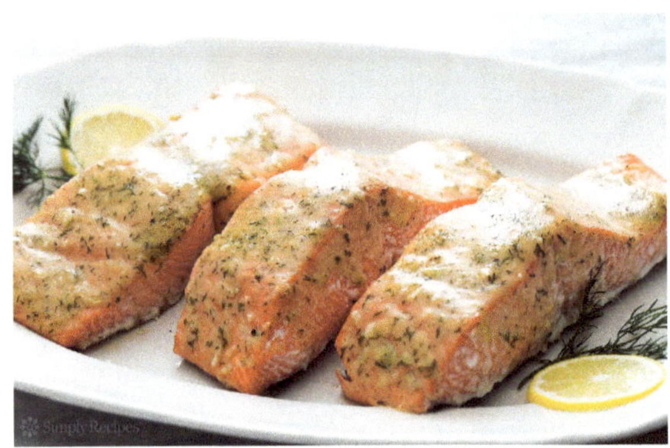

Ingredients:

- 5 ounces wild salmon
- 1 tsp. each of minced garlic and olive oil
- ½ tsp. Dijon mustard
- Juice from one-half lemon
- ½ tbsp. minced garlic
- 1 & 1/2 cup asparagus

Instructions:

1. Preheat your oven by setting it at 405 degrees Fahrenheit.
2. While preheating, get a bowl and mix lemon juice, olive oil, garlic, and mustard. This should serve as the marinade, which you need to pour over the salmon. Make sure that salmon is completely covered.
3. Get a baking sheet and arrange the salmon in there. Top it with lemon slices if you want. Put in your oven and bake for around ten to twelve minutes.
4. Prepare the asparagus spears and cut and remove their bottom stems.
5. Prepare a skillet and set it over medium-high heat. Spray it lightly with olive or coconut oil if you want.
6. Toss garlic and asparagus in the skillet. Sear them for around five minutes. Roll the asparagus to ensure that each side is seared.
7. The next step is plating the asparagus with the salmon. Serve.

Nutrition Facts:

Calories: 310

Protein: 33 grams

Fat: 14 grams

Carbs: 13 grams

Grilled Halibut with Avocado and Tomato Salsa

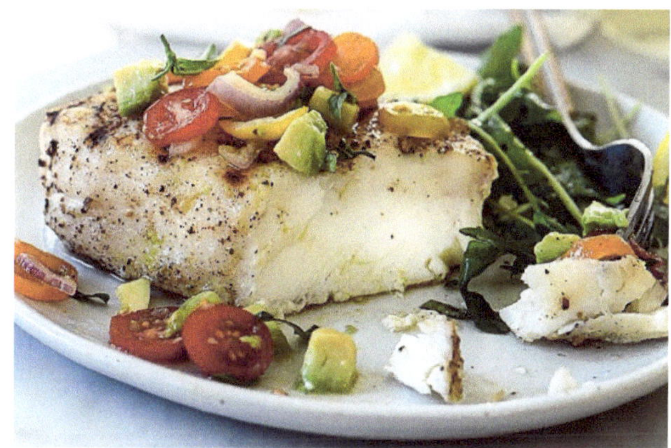

Ingredients:

- 2 pieces 6-oz. halibut filets
- Kosher salt
- Freshly ground black pepper
- Extra virgin olive oil
- Ingredients for the Salsa:
- 1 pint sliced heirloom cherry tomatoes
- ½ thinly sliced shallot
- 1 peeled, chopped and pitted avocado
- 1 tbsp. extra-virgin olive oil
- 2 sprigs slivered basil leaves
- Kosher salt
- Freshly ground black pepper
- 1 and ½ tsp. golden balsamic vinegar

Instructions:

1. Preheat your grill using high heat.
2. Use the olive oil to drizzle the halibut then season it with salt and pepper. Use grape-seed oil to oil the grates of the grill. Arrange the halibut filets in there. Make sure to press down the filet gently on the grate. Cook it on the grill until it easily flakes and is already opaque. It should take around five minutes per side.
3. Mix the cherry tomatoes, shallot, basil, and avocado together in a bowl. Do this while you are still waiting for the fish to cook.
4. Drizzle this mixture with golden balsamic vinegar and olive oil. Toss well to coat. Use some kosher salt and black pepper as seasonings.
5. Take the fish out of the grill once cooked then top it with the salsa you have created. Serve.

Nutrition Facts:

Calories: 256

Protein: 48 grams

Fat: 22 grams

Carbs: 14 grams

Shrimp Scampi

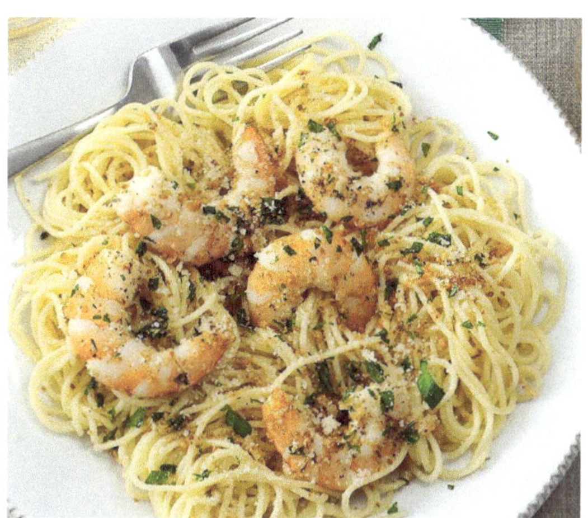

Ingredients:

- 2 tbsps. butter (unsalted)
- 8 ounces linguine
- 3 minced garlic cloves
- 1 lb. medium-sized peeled and deveined shrimp
- ¼ cup white wine
- ¼ tsp. red pepper flakes (crushed)
- ¼ cup lemon juice (freshly squeezed)
- Zest of 1 lemon
- ¼ cup Parmesan cheese (freshly grated)
- 2 tbsps. fresh parsley leaves (chopped)
- Kosher salt
- Freshly ground black pepper

Instructions:

1. Cook the pasta based on the instructions stated on its package. After cooking the pasta in boiling salted water, drain it well.
2. Prepare a large skillet then set it over medium-high heat. Melt butter in there. Cook garlic, red pepper flakes, and shrimp in the skillet while stirring occasionally. Do so until the mixture becomes pink. This should take around two to three minutes.
3. Pour lemon juice and add the wine. Season this mixture with salt and pepper. Simmer. Once done, take the skillet out of the heat. Stir in pasta and add the parsley and lemon zest. Mix well.

4. Garnish pasta with Parmesan cheese and serve right away.

Nutrition Facts:

Calories: 417

Carbs: 45.2 grams

Protein: 33 grams

Fat: 9.6 grams

Apple and Cinnamon Pork Chops

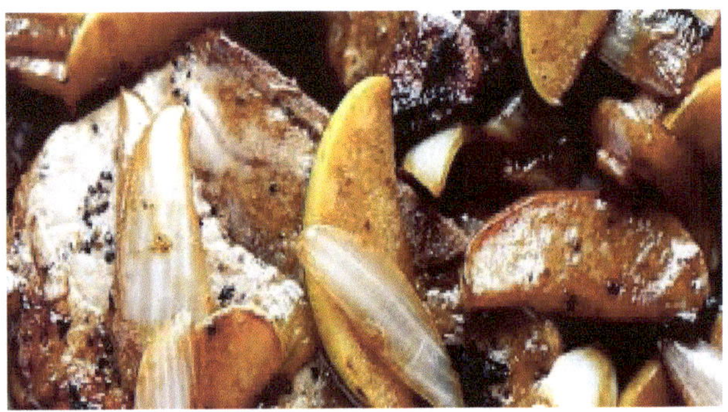

Ingredients:

- 4 rib-eye pork chops – around ¾-inch thick with bones
- 3 tbsps. divided butter
- Salt
- Pepper
- 2 tbsps. brown sugar (packed)
- 2 peeled, thinly sliced, and cored apples
- 1/3 cup heavy cream
- 2/3 cup apple cider vinegar
- 2 tsp. cinnamon (ground)
- 1 large halved onion (thinly sliced)
- A pinch of cayenne pepper (ground)

Instructions:

1. Season the pork chops generously with salt and pepper. Make sure to season the chops on two sides. Set them aside.
2. Melt butter in a skillet. Add the seasoned pork chops then cook them for around three minutes per side or until they turn brown. Put the pork chops on a plate and allow them to rest for around three minutes.

3. Put the skillet over medium-high heat. Melt one tablespoon of the butter in the skillet. Cook onion and apples there while stirring it occasionally for around five minutes or until the onion looks translucent. Add brown sugar, cayenne, and cinnamon.

4. The next ingredients you should add into the mixture are the cream and apple cider. After that, stir in the pork chops. Make sure that the pork chops are nestled into the liquid. Cook them until the pork's temperature is already 145 degrees Fahrenheit. Transfer the cooked pork chops on a plate.

5. Spoon the apple mixture on top of each pork chop and serve.

Nutrition Facts:

Calories: 555

Protein: 36 grams

Fat: 26 grams

Carbs: 20 grams

Beef Noodle Soup

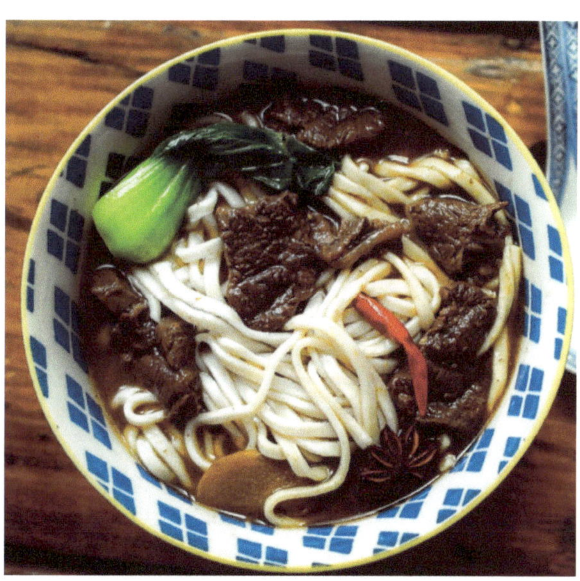

Ingredients:

- 2 cups beef broth (low-sodium)
- 1 lb. ground beef – Make sure it is lean.
- 1 cup finely diced celery stalk
- 1 cup of water
- 2 cups broccoli
- 1 cup sliced carrots
- 8 ounces canned bean sprouts
- ½ cup snow peas
- 2 cups whole-wheat pasta spaghetti
- 1 minced garlic clove

Instructions:

1. Set skillet over medium heat and cook beef until it turns brown.
2. Boil water and beef broth in a pot. Once it boils, stir in snow peas, celery, and carrots. Cook this mixture for around two to three minutes.
3. Add ground beef, bean sprouts, and broccoli next. Cook the mixture for one to two more minutes.
4. Stir in the pasta and garlic. Simmer for around eight minutes using low heat. Serve right away.

Nutrition Facts:

Calories: 394

Carbs: 42 grams

Protein: 31 grams

Fat: 11 grams

Chapter 6 – 6 Easy and Quick 30-Minute Snack Recipes for Bodybuilding

High-Protein Chicken Meatballs

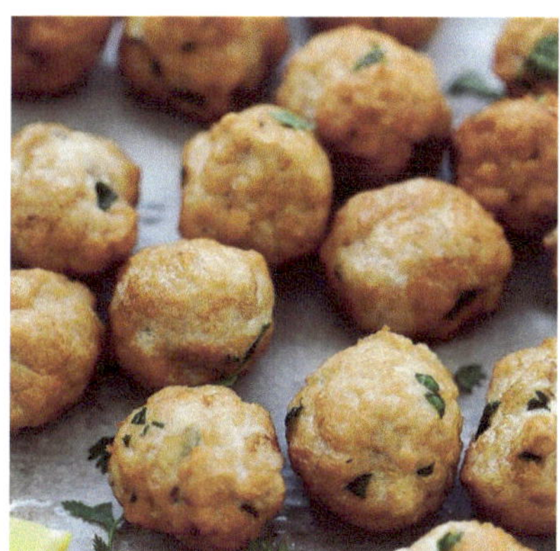

Ingredients:

- 90-gram rolled oats
- 1 lb. ground chicken
- 2 tsps. allspice
- 2 whole onions
- Salt
- Pepper

Instructions:

1. Set a pan on medium heat. Spray or grease the pan a bit to prevent the meatballs from sticking.
2. Chop or grate onions finely. Combine the finely grated onion with the remaining ingredients.
3. Form balls from this mixture. As much as possible, use a spoon when forming the balls to make the size consistent, which can also help in cooking them fast.
4. Fry the meatballs on the heated pan until cooked through. The meatballs should turn to golden brown before removing them from the pan.
5. Serve.

Nutrition Facts:

Calories: 519

Protein: 57 grams

Carbs: 32 grams

Fat: 15 grams

Grilled Chili Cheese Fries

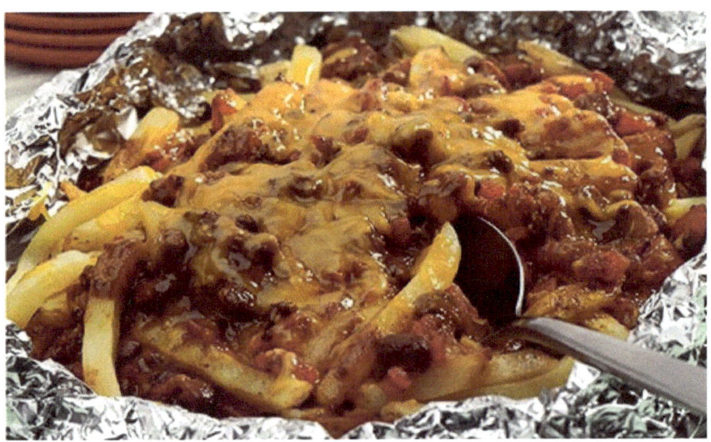

Ingredients:

- 1 bag steak fries
- 1 batch chili
- ½ cup cheddar cheese

Instructions:

1. Put a grill over medium heat.
2. While waiting for the grill to heat up, get a tin foil and arrange three to four thick pieces of it in layers. Each layer of tin foil should be on top of each other.
3. Put the fries in the middle part of the foil. Use the cheddar cheese and chili to top them.
4. You should then grill the fries with closed lid until the cheese melts and the fries become golden. This process should take around 25 to 30 minutes.
5. Serve.

Nutrition Facts:

Calories: 463

Carbs: 47 grams

Protein: 33 grams

Fat: 15 grams

Buffalo Chicken Sliders

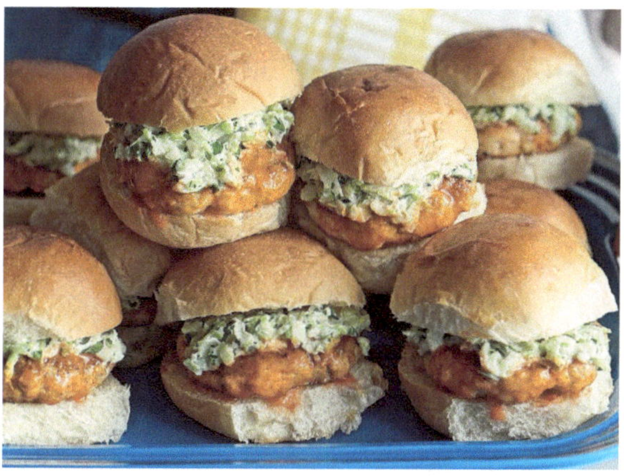

Ingredients:

- 2 lbs. skinless and boneless chicken breast – Make sure it is cooked and shredded, too.
- 1 pack of ranch dressing seasoning mix
- 1 cup wing sauce
- 12 slider buns
- ¼ cup blue cheese dressing (reduced fat)
- Some lettuce

Instructions:

1. Mix the chicken breast, ranch dressing, and wing sauce in a bowl. Toss well until the chicken breast is properly and evenly coated.
2. Put a lettuce leaf on every bun.
3. Use the shredded chicken mix as toppings.
4. Complete this snack recipe by adding a bit of blue cheese dressing on top. Serve right away.

Nutrition Facts:

Calories: 213

Protein: 20 grams

Carbs: 17 grams

Fat: 8 grams

Peanut Butter and Chocolate Chip French Toast

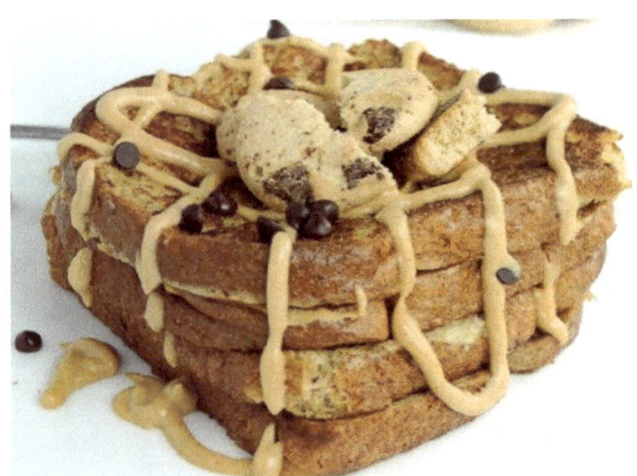

Ingredients:

- 4 slices of whole-wheat bread
- 1 tbsp. granulated sweetener
- ½ scoop of protein powder (vanilla-flavored)
- 2 whole eggs
- ½ tsp. cinnamon
- 2 tbsps. peanut butter
- ½ cup of milk
- 1 tsp. mini-chocolate chips

Instructions:

1. Preheat your griddle or pan using medium or high heat.
2. Mix egg, cinnamon, milk, and protein powder together.
3. Soak the bread slices one by one on the prepared egg mixture.

4. Cook the French toast on the heated griddle or pan for around 3 minutes per side. You will also know that it is already cooked if it is golden brown.
5. The next step is to heat the peanut butter until it melts. Drizzle it over the cooked French toast.
6. Sprinkle the chocolate chips on top then serve.

Nutrition Facts:

Calories: 450

Carbs: 46 grams

Protein: 40 grams

Fat: 13 grams

Egg White Bites

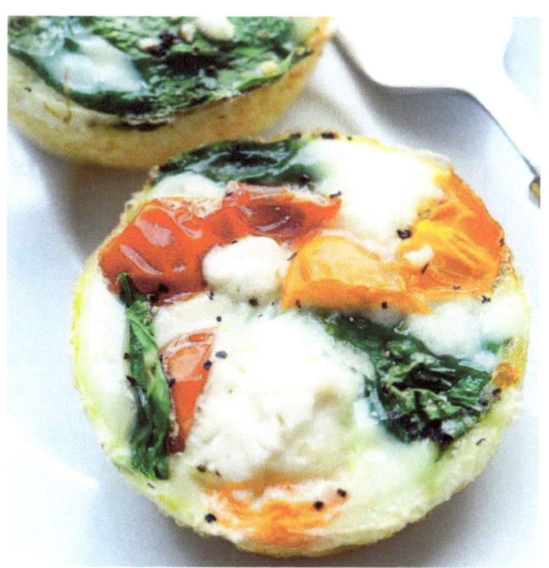

Ingredients:

- 10 egg whites
- 1 tsp. dried ground basil
- 1 finely diced whole onion
- 1 tomato
- 1 whole egg
- 1 dash black pepper

Instructions:

1. Whisk egg and the egg whites in a bowl.
2. Get a pan with 6 muffin tins. Pour equal amounts of the egg mixture into each tin.
3. Each portion should then be topped with one teaspoon each of the prepared onion and tomato. Use the black pepper and basil as toppings, too.
4. Bake in your oven for around 8 minutes or when your preferred doneness is reached.
5. Serve.

Nutrition Facts:

Calories: 48

Protein: 7 grams

Carbs: 3 grams

Fat: 1 gram

Oatmeal and Tuna Pancakes

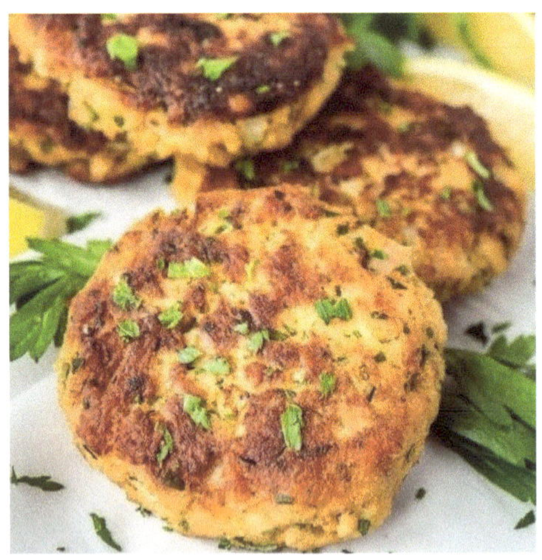

Ingredients:

- 2 eggs
- 1 can of tuna

- 1 onion
- 4 tbsps. oatmeal
- Olive oil
- 1 tsp. mustard

Instructions:

1. Drain tuna.
2. Add eggs, chopped onion, mustard, and oatmeal into it. Combine the ingredients well until they are well-mixed.
3. Heat a pan then add olive oil on it. Begin forming pancakes from the created mixture while waiting for the oil to heat up a bit.
4. Fry both sides of the pancakes. You will know that they are cooked when each side turns to golden brown.
5. Serve. It would be best to serve it together with yogurt, parsley, and fresh tomatoes.

Nutrition Facts:

Calories: 410

Protein: 43 grams

Carbs: 30 grams

Fat: 14 grams

Chapter 7 – 6 Easy and Quick 30-Minute Dessert Recipes for Bodybuilding

Peanut Butter Tofu Pudding

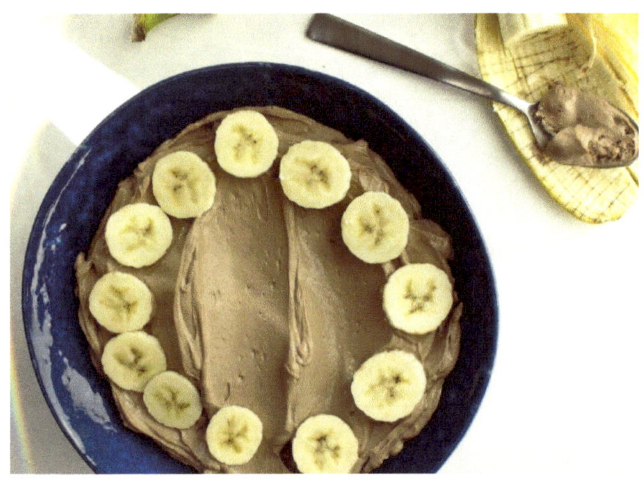

Ingredients:

- 2 blocks of extra-firm and drained tofu (14 ounces each)
- 2 eggs – You may also use half a cup of milk as a substitute for eggs.
- ½ cup of cocoa powder
- ¾ cup crunchy or smooth peanut butter
- 7 tbsps. honey
- Sliced banana

Instructions:

1. Place the two blocks of tofu in between two large-sized plates. Get a large bowl with a heavy item on it and put it on top of the plates. You have to do this to weigh down the tofu and remove any excess moisture. It should take around five minutes.
2. Blend peanut butter, eggs, tofu, honey, and cocoa powder in your blender using high speed. Scrape down the sides every now and then while blending.

Continue doing this until it shows a smooth consistency. You know that the pudding is done if it is also already extremely creamy.

3. Refrigerate then serve. It would be best to serve this pudding with sliced banana.

Nutrition Facts:

Calories: 299

Carbs: 30 grams

Fat: 18 grams

Protein: 10 grams

Peanut Butter Donuts with Glaze

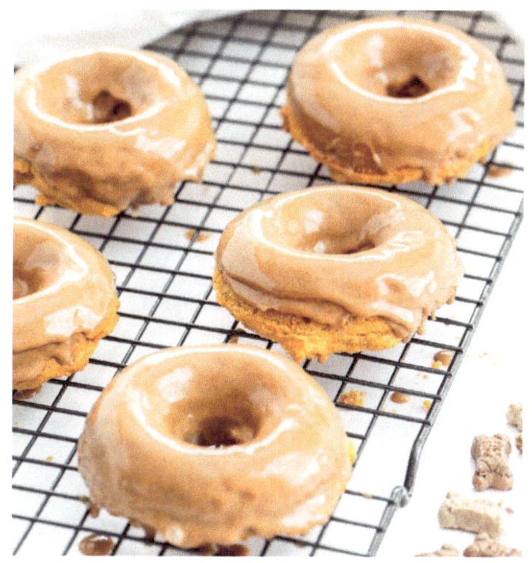

Ingredients:

- 2/3 cup milk
- 1 tsp. each of vanilla extract and apple cider vinegar
- 1 cup all-purpose flour
- 3 tbsps. coconut oil
- 1 and ¼ tsp. table salt
- 1 scoop whey protein powder (oatmeal cookie flavor
- 1 and ½ tsp. baking powder

- Ingredients for the Glaze:
- 1 tbsp. coconut oil
- ¼ cup peanut butter

Instructions:

1. Preheat your oven. Get a donut pan and grease it.
2. Mix milk, oil, vanilla, and vinegar in a small-sized bowl well. Get another bowl and mix flour, salt, whey powder, and baking powder in there. Whisk well.
3. Mix the wet and dry ingredients until you notice the batter coming together. Pour it right away into the donut pan.
4. Bake for around 15 minutes or until it gets into your desired doneness. After that, take the baked donuts out of the oven and let them cool down.
5. Prepare the glaze by putting the coconut oil and peanut butter mixture in the microwave for 30 seconds. Mix until it becomes smooth.
6. Dip the cooked and cooled donuts into the prepared glaze. After that, put the glazed donuts on a wire rack and let them set.
7. Serve.

Nutrition Facts:

Calories: 264

Carbs: 21 grams

Fat: 16 grams

Protein: 10 grams

Pumpkin Spice Protein Cookies

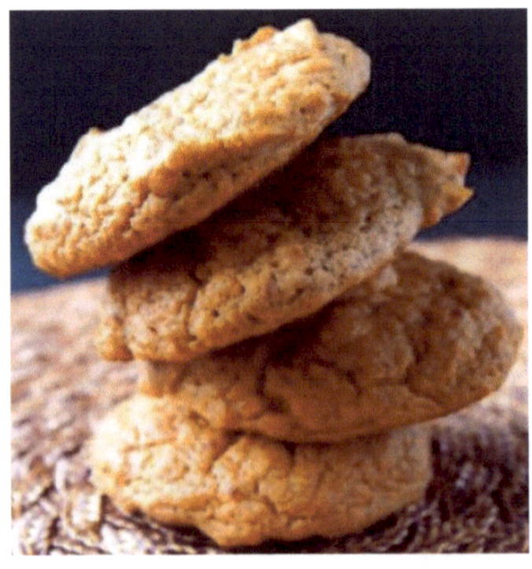

Ingredients:

- ¼ cup egg whites
- 1/3 cup pumpkin puree
- 1 cup white kidney beans
- 37 grams of strawberries (freeze-dried)
- 1 scoop of vanilla chai protein powder
- 1 tsp. each of baking powder, pumpkin pie spice, and vanilla extract

Instructions:

1. Preheat your oven.
2. Blend the beans in your food processor until the texture becomes smooth.
3. Add the other ingredients into the food processor. Blend until the mixture becomes smoother and well-mixed.
4. Form ten circles from the blended batter and arrange them in a parchment paper-lined baking sheet.
5. Put the baking sheet in your oven. Bake the cookies for ten to twelve minutes.
6. Once done, you can take the baking sheet out of the oven. Transfer the cookies on a wire rack to cool down before serving.

Nutrition Facts:

Calories: 78

Carbs: 11 grams

Protein: 7 grams

Fat: 1 gram

Peanut Butter and Chocolate Mug Cake

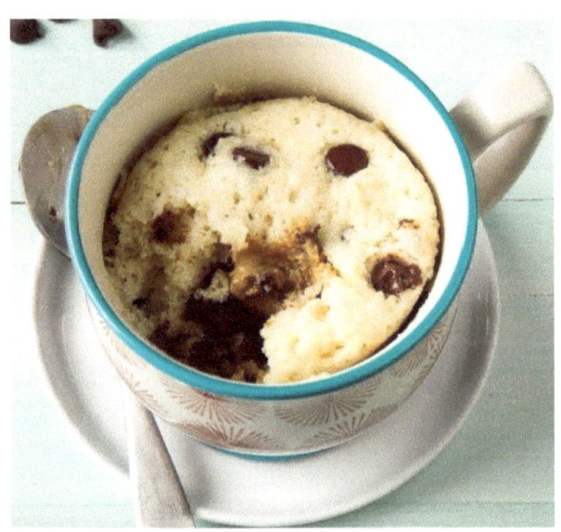

Ingredients:

- ¼ cup chocolate-powdered peanut butter
- 1 scoop chocolate delight protein powder
- 1 tbsp. unsweetened cocoa powder
- 1 whole egg
- ¼ tsp. baking powder
- 2 tbsps. almond milk
- 1/3 cup applesauce (unsweetened)
- ½ tbsp. vanilla extract

Ingredients for the Frosting:

- 2 tbsps. non-fat milk
- 3 tbsps. peanut butter (powdered)

Instructions:

1. Mix all the dry ingredients in one bowl.
2. Get another bowl then whisk the egg. Stir in the almond milk, vanilla extract, and applesauce.
3. Fold the mixed dry ingredients into the wet. Get a couple of mugs and spray it with some cooking spray. Pour the batter mixture into both bowls.
4. Each mug cake should then be microwaved for around ninety seconds.

5. You should then take it out of the microwave. Let the cakes cool down while you are mixing the required ingredients for the frosting.
6. Once the cakes cool down, top them with the frosting. Serve.

Nutrition Facts:

Calories: 296

Protein: 25 grams

Carbs: 24 grams

Fat: 11 grams

Simple Brownie with Banana and Yogurt

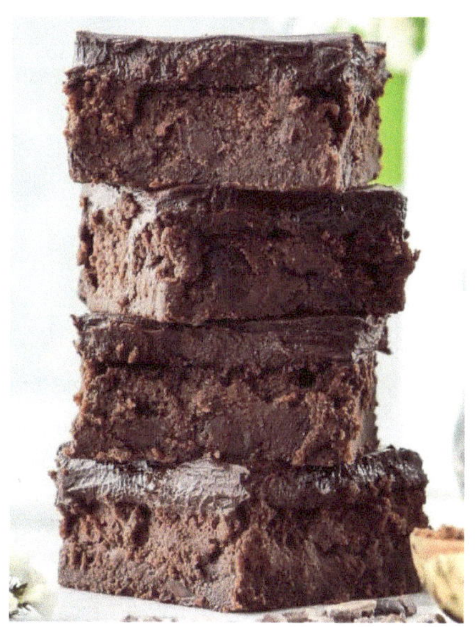

Ingredients:

- ¼ cup plain Greek yogurt (non-fat)
- ½ of one banana
- 1 scoop chocolate delight protein powder
- 1/8 tsp. baking powder
- ½ tbsp. unsweetened cocoa powder

- 2 tbsps. almond flour

Instructions:

1. Mash banana in a bowl.
2. Add the protein powder, Greek yogurt, baking powder, almond flour, and cocoa powder. Stir well.
3. Spray non-stick cooking oil into individual-squared ramekin. Pour the mixture into the ramekin. You may also use a mug if you do not have a ramekin.
4. Microwave it for around one and a half to two minutes. Sprinkle some confectioner's sugar on top then serve.

Nutrition Facts:

Calories: 275

Protein: 27 grams

Carbs: 26 grams

Fat: 7 grams

Blueberry Protein Cake

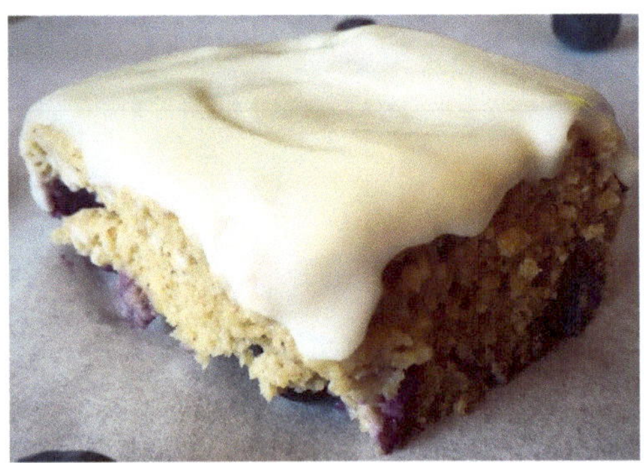

Ingredients:

- 1/3 cup blueberries
- ¼ cup applesauce (unsweetened)
- 2 egg whites
- 1 scoop of vanilla chai protein powder
- 2 tbsps. each of coconut flour and ground flaxseed
- 1/8 tsp. baking powder
- 2 tbsps. almond milk

Ingredients for the Frosting:

- ¼ scoop vanilla chai protein powder
- 2 ounces Greek yogurt (plain and non-fat)

Instructions:

1. Blend egg whites, applesauce, coconut flour, flaxseed meal, baking powder, almond milk, and protein powder in a blender.
2. Add the blueberries.
3. Pour this mixture into a small bowl, mug, or ramekin.
4. Microwave the mixture for two minutes.
5. Wait for the cake to cool down. While doing so, you can mix protein powder and Greek yogurt.
6. Use this mixture to top each cake then serve.

Nutrition Facts:

Calories: 376

Protein: 38 grams

Carbs: 35 grams

Fat: 9 grams

Chapter 8 – 5 Common Mistakes Beginners Make when Preparing their Bodybuilding Diet Meals

If you are still a beginner in bodybuilding, then you have to make sure that your regular exercises are paired up with the right diet. You have to understand how to prepare meals that perfectly suit your bodybuilding journey.

To help you out, here is a compilation of the most common mistakes beginners make when preparing their bodybuilding diet meals. Avoid them as much as possible so you will have higher chances of achieving your target.

#1 – Not including sodium

A lot of beginners in bodybuilding believe that salt/sodium should not be taken at all as it might only cause excess water retention. This belief led them to let go of all those foods that contain any amount of salt. However, you should not completely eliminate sodium from your diet.

It is because it helps a lot in regulating the fluid balance of your body. Too little consumption of sodium might also initiate water retention, which is supposed to be what you want to avoid. Aside from that, an extremely low level of sodium can have a negative effect on your muscle and nerve function.

It can even trigger muscle weakness and cramps. With that in mind, make some adjustments into your daily bodybuilding diet and try to include moderate quantity of sodium. It can contribute to preventing muscle cramps plus it helps you stick to your diet since it adds more taste and flavor to your food.

#2 – Cutting down on carbs excessively

Another mistake that you should avoid is cutting down carbs excessively. Yes, reducing your carb intake can help you lose weight and achieve your target body.

However, you should avoid reducing it too much to the point that your diet already has zero or only trace amounts of it.

If you cut it down too much, then you may end up looking too lean, meaning you get too much leaner than what you had initially expected. It is because insufficient carbs in your body might cause it to go into starvation mode. It can cause your muscles to start burning their own protein to produce energy.

Cut down on carbs but make sure your body still receives its daily recommended requirement of it.

#3 – Yo-yo dieting

You should also avoid yo-yo dieting if you want to gain the best results from bodybuilding. Yo-yo dieting usually involves going from one extreme habit to another through calorie consumption. For example, there are days in a particular week when you overly restrict your calorie intake followed by days when you overeat.

It could also be that you tend to make up for certain mistakes, like overeating or being unable to stick to a nutrition plan the previous day, by significantly cutting calories or increasing calorie expenditure. You have to avoid this mistake as much as possible as it might only lead to the development of an unbreakable and vicious cycle. It might also cause you to build a poor relationship with foods.

Instead of going to the extreme to correct what you did that causes you to fall off your nutrition or meal plans, just try to get back to the habit normally. Don't overburden yourself with negative feelings, like guilt, as it might only lead to drastic actions that involve your intake of calories. What you should do, instead, is to focus on sticking to your meal plans from now on.

#4 – Extremely low-calorie intake for a prolonged period

One way to lose excess body fats is to eat few calories. However, this fact also causes some bodybuilders and dieters to go to the extreme by sticking to a meal plan, which is extremely low on calories for a long period, months to years, even. Note that sticking to an extreme diet is already stressful for the body.

If you combine it with intense exercises, particularly those performed by bodybuilders, then you will be at risk of developing a high level of cortisol, a stress hormone, for an extended period. The problem is that an excessively high cortisol level might lead to a significant increase in your blood sugar.

One way to avoid this problem is to take a break of one to two weeks after you were able to retain an intense calorie deficit after six weeks. Note that no matter how short your break is from dieting, it is already helpful in your metabolism plus it can greatly improve your gym performance, making your bodybuilding efforts produce better results.

#5 – Insufficient protein intake

Make sure that your bodybuilding diet also gives you your body the amount of protein it needs every day. If you want to gain lean muscles, then make sure to monitor your daily protein intake. It should be at least one gram for every pound of bodyweight. Never underestimate the importance of protein-rich foods in your bodybuilding journey.

Make sure, however, that most of the protein that your body receives comes from whole food sources. These include red meat, turkey, chicken, fish, eggs, cheese, and Greek yogurt.

By avoiding these mistakes, you can definitely prepare your meals in accordance with your bodybuilding efforts as well as the results you desire to achieve.

Bonus Chapter – 1-day Meal Plan to Kick Start your Bodybuilding Journey

As a bonus, here is a 1-day bodybuilding meal plan that you should consider using as your guide when preparing your meals.

Breakfast	Mid-morning Snack	Lunch (Pre-workout)	Post-workout Snack	Dinner
2 boiled eggs 1 banana	Natural yogurt 1 kiwi (sliced) with chia seeds as toppings	Grilled cheese sandwich with lettuce, cucumbers, tomatoes, and olives	Chocolate protein shake	Rice and veggies Chicken breast

Conclusion

Bodybuilding is all about building muscles and making them as lean as possible. It is not only all about athletic performance. You can't get the results you want from bodybuilding, though, if you don't combine your regular exercises with special attention to your daily diet.

When preparing your diet, pay close attention to what your body specifically needs. Ensure that it includes nutrient-dense foods. Make sure that your body gets enough protein, too. Aside from that, remember that your bodybuilding efforts will only produce favorable results if you restrict your intake of unhealthy foods, like deep-fried ones as well as those rich in sugar.

Your goal is to make your body receive all the nutrients it needs to build muscle and improve your overall health. Hopefully, the information in this book, as well as the bodybuilding recipes we have provided, can help you reach your health and fitness goals.

-- [Gabriel Buchanan]

Unit Conversion Table

53

COOKING CONVERSION CHART

Measurement

CUP	ONCES	MILLILITERS	TABLESPOONS
8 cup	64 oz	1895 ml	128
6 cup	48 oz	1420 ml	96
5 cup	40 oz	1180 ml	80
4 cup	32 oz	960 ml	64
2 cup	16 oz	480 ml	32
1 cup	8 oz	240 ml	16
3/4 cup	6 oz	177 ml	12
2/3 cup	5 oz	158 ml	11
1/2 cup	4 oz	118 ml	8
3/8 cup	3 oz	90 ml	6
1/3 cup	2.5 oz	79 ml	5.5
1/4 cup	2 oz	59 ml	4
1/8 cup	1 oz	30 ml	3
1/16 cup	1/2 oz	15 ml	1

Temperature

FAHRENHEIT	CELSIUS
100 °F	37 °C
150 °F	65 °C
200 °F	93 °C
250 °F	121 °C
300 °F	150 °C
325 °F	160 °C
350 °F	180 °C
375 °F	190 °C
400 °F	200 °C
425 °F	220 °C
450 °F	230 °C
500 °F	260 °C
525 °F	274 °C
550 °F	288 °C

Weight

IMPERIAL	METRIC
1/2 oz	15 g
1 oz	29 g
2 oz	57 g
3 oz	85 g
4 oz	113 g
5 oz	141 g
6 oz	170 g
8 oz	227 g
10 oz	283 g
12 oz	340 g
13 oz	369 g
14 oz	397 g
15 oz	425 g
1 lb	453 g